MASTERING HAND REFLEXOLOGY TECHNIQUES

Notice The Healing Potential of Your Hands

John J. Elliot

TABLE OF CONTENTS

CHAPTER 1: INTRODUCTION TO HAND REFLEXOLOGY

- What is Reflexology?
- History and Origins of Reflexology
- Benefits of Hand Reflexology
- Differences Between Hand and Foot Reflexology

CHAPTER 2: UNDERSTANDING THE BASICS

- Anatomy of the Hand
- Key Reflex Points on the Hand
- How Reflexology Works

CHAPTER 3: PREPARATION AND PRECAUTIONS

- Contraindications and Safety Considerations
- Preparing Yourself and the Client
- Setting Up the Treatment Space

- Hygiene and Sanitation

CHAPTER 4: HAND REFLEXOLOGY TECHNIQUES

- Basic Techniques: Thumb Walking, Finger Walking, and Pressure Techniques
- Advanced Techniques: Rotations, Hooking, and Point Pressing
- Using Tools and Aids

CHAPTER 5: THE REFLEX ZONES OF THE HAND

- Zone Therapy Theory
- Detailed Maps of Hand Reflex Zones
- Understanding Reflex Points for Each Body System

CHAPTER 6: STEP-BY-STEP HAND REFLEXOLOGY ROUTINE

- Warm-Up Exercises and Relaxation Techniques

CHAPTER 9: COMBINING HAND REFLEXOLOGY WITH OTHER PRACTICES

- Aromatherapy
- Acupressure and Acupuncture
- Massage Therapy
- Mindfulness and Meditation

CHAPTER 10: SELF-CARE AND MAINTENANCE

- Self-Reflexology Techniques
- Daily Hand Care Tips
- Exercises to Enhance Hand Flexibility and Strength

CHAPTER 11: CASE STUDIES AND TESTIMONIALS

- Real-Life Case Studies
- Success Stories from Practitioners and Clients

CHAPTER 12: BECOMING A PROFESSIONAL REFLEXOLOGIST

CHAPTER 1

INTRODUCTION TO HAND REFLEXOLOGY

What is reflexology?

Reflexology is a therapeutic treatment based on the idea that certain points on the feet, hands, and ears connect to distinct sections of the body. Reflexologists think that applying pressure to these locations can improve health and well-being in the relevant organs and systems. The fundamental idea is that these spots, or "reflex zones," are energetically linked to various regions of the body and that activating them may clear blockages, restore balance, and improve general health.

Reflexology is sometimes mistaken for massage, although the two are separate therapies. Massage manipulates muscles and tissues to reduce tension and promote relaxation, whereas reflexology concentrates on particular reflex sites to alter the body's internal systems. The reflexologist targets these reflex areas with particular procedures such as thumb walking, finger walking, and acupressure.

Reflexology has several benefits. Many individuals utilize reflexology to relieve tension, discomfort, increase circulation, and promote relaxation. It is also used to treat certain health problems like headaches, intestinal disorders, and hormone abnormalities. Reflexology is a holistic therapy, which means it takes into account the entire person's mind, body, and spiritand seeks to enhance total well-being rather than treating individual problems in isolation.
Several hypotheses support reflexology's efficacy. One of the leading explanations is that it stimulates the neurological system. The concept is that pushing on reflex points delivers messages from the peripheral nervous system to the central nervous system, causing a relaxation response and reducing tension. Another idea holds that reflexology works by balancing the body's energy, similar to the concepts of acupuncture and traditional Chinese kk, in which

the flow of "qi" or life force energy is critical for health.

Scientific study on reflexology is ongoing, and while some studies have yielded promising outcomes, others ask for more rigorous trials to definitively determine its usefulness. Nonetheless, many patients claim considerable advantages from frequent reflexology sessions, and it is still a popular supplementary therapy across the world.

Reflexology is not a replacement for traditional medical therapy, but rather a complimentary technique that may be used with other treatments. It's especially tempting to people who choose non-invasive, drug-free treatments. As with any therapeutic technique, it is critical to visit with a knowledgeable reflexologist and confirm that they are appropriately educated and certified.

To summarize, reflexology is a total approach that employs particular techniques to stimulate reflex sites on the hands, feet and ears to improve health and wellness. While its processes are still being studied, its effects on stress relief, pain reduction and overall relaxation make it an important tool in the field of complementary and alternative medicine.

History and Origins of Reflexology

The history of reflexology is broad and varied, with origins dating back to ancient cultures. Evidence indicates that reflexology has been performed for thousands of years, with different civilizations establishing their procedures and ideas regarding the body's reflex zones.
One of the first records of a reflexology-like technique dates back to ancient Egypt. A tomb artwork from around 2330 BCE displays what looks to be a reflexology therapy. The picture, discovered in the tomb of an Egyptian physician called Ankhmahor, depicts two individuals getting treatment for their hands and feet. The hieroglyphic writings surrounding the artwork indicate that the practice was intended to promote health and well-being.

Similarly, reflexology has been practiced in ancient China from roughly 2700 BCE. Chinese medicine has long highlighted the importance of energy flow, or "qi," and how it affects health. The Chinese created detailed maps of the body's energy lines, or meridians, which contain particular spots on the hands and feet that correlate to different organs and systems. This old understanding provided the foundation for current reflexology procedures.

In India, reflexology is linked to the ancient therapeutic tradition of Ayurveda, which dates back over 5,000 years. Ayurvedic practitioners massage and apply pressure to the feet to balance the body's energies and promote healing. Ayurvedic teachings stress the interdependence of the body, mind and spirit, which reflects reflexology's holistic approach.

The contemporary evolution of reflexology as we know it now dates back to the early twentieth century. Dr. William Fitzgerald, an American ear, nose, and throat doctor, is widely recognized for bringing reflexology to the Western world. He created a method called "zone therapy," which split the body into 10 vertical zones. Fitzgerald observed that applying pressure to certain areas inside these zones might have a healing impact on the relevant sections of the body. His work established the contemporary practice of reflexology.

In the 1930s and 1940s, **Eunice Ingham**, a nurse and physiotherapist, improved and popularized reflexology. **Ingham** is widely regarded as the mother of modern reflexology, having mapped out comprehensive reflex spots on the feet and hands and associated them with particular organs and systems. Her publications, "Stories the Feet Can Tell" and "Stories the Feet Have Told," were essential works in the area, raising awareness and knowledge of reflexology.

Reflexology continued to evolve during the twentieth century, with practitioners all around the world contributing to its advancement. Reflexology is now widely practiced across the world and acknowledged as an alternative therapy that can improve general health and well-being. Professional organizations and certification systems have been developed to guarantee that reflexologists maintain high levels of training and practice.

The history of reflexology demonstrates humanity's ongoing pursuit of holistic healing techniques. From the ancient Egyptians and Chinese to current practitioners, reflexology has been respected for its ability to improve well-being via the simple but profound act of activating reflex spots on the hands and feet. As research advances and our awareness of the body's connection grows, reflexology is an important and expanding topic in complementary and alternative medicine.

Benefits of Hand Reflexology

Hand reflexology, a treatment based on ancient therapeutic traditions, has several advantages for physical, emotional, and mental health. This supplementary therapy consists of applying pressure to particular locations on the hands that correspond to various organs and systems in the body. Here are some of the major advantages of hand reflexology:

1. **Stress Reduction and Relaxation:** One of the most noticeable advantages of hand reflexology is its ability to promote relaxation and relieve tension. Pressure applied to reflex sites can activate the parasympathetic nervous system, resulting in a sense of calm and relaxation. This technique reduces tension and anxiety, which are frequent in today's fast-paced society. Reflexology reduces stress and lowers cortisol levels, which improves general health.

2. **Improved Circulation:** Hand reflexology can help improve blood circulation throughout the body. The pressure tactics employed during a session increase blood flow, which helps to deliver oxygen and critical nutrients to cells more efficiently. Improved circulation also helps to remove toxins and waste products from the

body, which promotes detoxification and boosts overall vigor.

3. **Pain Relief:** Another key advantage of hand reflexology is the possibility of pain treatment. Practitioners can assist relieve pain from a variety of diseases, including headaches, arthritis, and carpal tunnel syndrome, by focusing on certain reflex points. Reflexology works by blocking pain pathways and increasing the production of endorphins, the body's natural painkillers.

4. **Enhanced Immune Function:** Regular hand reflexology treatments help strengthen the immune system, making it more resistant to infections and diseases. Reflexology stimulates reflex sites involved with the lymphatic system and other immune-related organs, which helps to boost the body's natural defensive systems. This increased immune activity can reduce the frequency and severity of common illnesses such as colds and flu.

5. Improved digestive health: Hand reflexology can help improve digestive health by activating reflex sites associated with the stomach, intestines, and other digestive organs. This stimulation can assist to normalize bowel motions, decrease bloating, and relieve gastrointestinal symptoms. For anyone suffering from persistent digestive disorders, reflexology provides a natural and non-invasive way to improve digestive function.

6. **Enhanced mental clarity and focus:** Hand reflexology's soothing benefits extend beyond physical well-being. Reflexology can increase mental clarity and attention by lowering tension and increasing relaxation. Individuals frequently report feeling more focused and alert following a session, making it an important tool for those who require high levels of cognitive function in their everyday lives.

7. **Better Sleep Quality:** Hand reflexology can greatly enhance sleep quality by encouraging calm and lowering anxiety. Many people

experience sleep difficulties as a result of stress and a hyperactive mind. Reflexology relaxes the nervous system, making it simpler to fall and remain asleep. Improved sleep quality promotes general health and well-being.

8. **Emotional Balance:** Hand reflexology can also improve emotional well-being. The exercise helps to balance the body's energy, which can improve emotional health. By treating underlying stress and tension, reflexology can help people feel more balanced and emotionally stable.

Finally, hand reflexology has several advantages that might improve physical, emotional, and mental wellness. Its capacity to promote relaxation, enhance circulation, reduce pain, increase immunological function, and support general well-being makes it an excellent supplementary therapy. Hand reflexology, whether used alone or in combination with other therapies, offers a natural and comprehensive approach to improving health.

Differences in Hand and Foot Reflexology:

Reflexology is a therapeutic therapy that includes applying pressure to certain spots on the hands or feet, each representing a different organ or system in the body. While hand and foot reflexology have similar underlying principles, there are significant differences between the two practices. Understanding these distinctions can help people select the best type of reflexology for their needs.

1. **Accessibility and Convenience:** One of the most important distinctions between hand and foot reflexology is accessibility. Hand reflexology can be performed easily and discreetly almost anywhere, making it ideal for people with busy schedules. Hand reflexology allows you to practice anywhere, including at work, on public transportation, or at home, without the need for any special equipment or conditions. Foot reflexology, on the other hand, typically requires a more relaxed setting in

which the individual can comfortably remove their shoes and socks, making it less convenient in some situations.

2. **Sensitivity and pain thresholds:** The hands and feet have different sensitivity and pain thresholds. Hand reflexology is less sensitive than foot reflexology, making it a more comfortable option for people who have a low pain threshold or find foot reflexology too intense. However, the feet have a higher concentration of nerve endings, making foot reflexology more effective in stimulating specific reflex points. Individuals with sensitive feet may choose hand reflexology to alleviate pain.

3. **Scope of Reflex Points:** Both the hands and feet have reflex sites that relate to the whole body, albeit the mapping of these points varies significantly. Foot reflexology is frequently seen as more complete because of the increased surface area of the foot, which allows for more exact targeting of reflex sites. The hands have a

decreased surface area, making it difficult to detect and stimulate specific spots with the same precision. Despite this, hand reflexology can still successfully address a wide range of health concerns.

4. **Techniques and Pressure Application:** The procedures utilized in hand and foot reflexology might vary because of the anatomical variances between the hands and feet. In hand reflexology, practitioners commonly use their thumbs and fingers to apply pressure, adopting techniques such as thumb walking and finger walking. Foot reflexology may entail extra procedures like knuckle rolling or utilizing specialized instruments to deliver deeper pressure. The diversity in procedures reflects the specific qualities of each place, guaranteeing that the most effective ways are applied for the best outcomes.

5. **Conditions Treated:** While both hand and foot reflexology can address a number of health concerns, certain illnesses may react better to

one type over the other. For instance, hand reflexology is particularly effective for diseases affecting the upper body, such as headaches, neck discomfort, and respiratory disorders, due to the closeness of reflex sites on the hands to these areas. Because of the location of comparable reflex sites on the feet, foot reflexology is frequently more beneficial for lower body ailments such as digestive disorders, lower back discomfort, and reproductive health.

6. **Practitioner Preferences and Client Comfort:** Practitioners may select hand or foot reflexology depending on their training, expertise, and the requirements of their customers. Client comfort is also an important issue. Some people may feel more at ease with hand reflexology, particularly if they are self-conscious about their feet or have foot-related ailments such as athlete's foot or plantar wart. Others may find foot reflexology more calming and helpful.

7. **Integration of Other Therapies:** Hand and foot reflexology can be used with other therapeutic approaches, however the choice may vary depending on the nature of the therapy. Hand reflexology may be readily coupled with techniques such as aromatherapy since essential oils can be administered to the hands without discomfort. Foot reflexology complements techniques such as foot baths and pedicures, which improves the whole therapeutic experience.

In conclusion, while hand and foot reflexology have similar fundamental principles, they differ in terms of accessibility, sensitivity, reflex point scope, methodologies, ailments addressed, practitioner choice, and integration with other treatments. Understanding these distinctions can assist individuals and practitioners in selecting the most effective kind of reflexology to attain the desired health results.

CHAPTER 2

ANATOMY OF HAND

The human hand is a complicated structure made up of bones, muscles, tendons, ligaments, and nerves that all work together to complete various movements and jobs. Understanding the anatomy of the hand is essential for successful reflexology therapy.

Bones and Joint:

The hand is made up of 27 bones, which are classified into three groups: carpals, metacarpals, and phalanges.

Carpal Bones: The wrist has eight (8) carpal bones grouped in two rows. These little, oddly formed bones form a solid but flexible foundation for the hand.

The palm has five (5) metacarpal bones, one for each finger. These bones are essential for hand strength and mobility.

Each finger has three (3) phalanges (proximal, middle, and distal), except the thumb, which only has two. These bones allow finger flexion and extension.

Muscles and Tendons:

The hand muscles are classified as intrinsic and extrinsic;

Intrinsic Muscles: These muscles are found within the hand itself. They govern fine motor movements and include the thenar and hypothenar muscles (for thumb and small finger motions), as well as the interossei and lumbrical muscles (for finger movements).

Extrinsic muscles: These muscles begin in the forearm and extend to the hand. They regulate large motor movements and are in charge of strong grabbing and lifting activities.

Tendons link muscles and bones, allowing muscular contractions to move them. The flexor tendons on the palm side permit finger flexion, whereas the extensor tendons on the back of the hand allow finger extension.

Nerves and Blood vessels:

Three major nerves innervate the hand:

Median nerve: The thumb, index, middle, and portion of the ring fingers are all controlled median nerves. It is essential for a precise grip and fine motor abilities.

Ulnar Nerve: Controls the little finger and a portion of the ring finger. It is essential for power gripping and hand strength.

The radial nerve: It controls the back of the hand and gives feeling to the thumb side.
The radial and ulnar arteries provide blood to the hand, ensuring that all tissues receive oxygen and nutrients.

Ligaments and Joints:

Ligaments link bones and provide support to joints. The hand contains numerous major joints.

The carpometacarpal joints connect the carpal and metacarpal bones.
Metacarpophalangeal joints connect the metacarpal bones to the proximal phalanges, allowing the fingers to flex and extend.
Interphalangeal joints are located between the phalanges and allow for delicate finger motions.

Skin and Sensory receptors:

The skin of our palms is thick and includes multiple sensory receptors that allow us to experience textures, temperatures, and pain. These receptors are essential for hand reflexology because they enable practitioners to detect minute changes and reactions in the tissues.

To summarize, the hand's architecture is complex and precisely adjusted, allowing for a vast variety of actions and functions. Understanding this intricacy is critical for anybody practicing hand reflexology since it allows them to execute treatments correctly and efficiently, enhancing therapeutic effects.

Key Reflex Points in the Hand

Reflexology of the hand works on the concept that certain locations on the hand connect to different sections of the body. By stimulating these reflex sites, you can encourage healing and balance in the associated regions. We'll look at the most important reflex spots on the hand and how they relate to other regions of the body.

Head and Brain Reflex Points:

Thumb: The thumb symbolizes the head and intellect. The tip of the thumb belongs to the brain, whereas the region around the base of the thumb is associated with the neck and throat.

Stimulating these regions may help relieve headaches, migraines and neck stress.

Spinal Reflex Points: The spine is represented by the inside border of the thumb, which extends down to the wrist. This region, which extends from the thumb tip (cervical spine) to the wrist (sacral spine), can be massaged to ease back discomfort and promote spinal health.

Digestive System Reflex Points: The digestive organs, which include the stomach, liver, intestines, and pancreas, are located in the center of the palm. Massaging this region can help with digestion, stomach discomfort, and liver function.

Respiratory System Reflex Points: The base of the thumb, located on the palm side, is related to the respiratory system, which includes the lungs and bronchial tubes. Stimulating this region helps alleviate respiratory problems such as asthma, bronchitis, and colds.

Heart and Circulatory Reflex Points: The cardiac reflex point is placed in the middle of the left palm. Massaging this region can help with heart health, circulation, and the symptoms of cardiovascular disease.

Kidney and Urinary System Reflex Points: The kidneys and bladder are represented at the base of both hands' little fingers. Stimulating these areas can assist the body in cleansing, maintaining kidney function, and relieving urinary tract problems.

Endocrine System Reflex Points: The fingertips, particularly the pads of each finger, correspond to the endocrine glands, which include the pituitary, thyroid, and adrenal glands. Massage these points can help to balance hormones and improve overall endocrine function.

Lymphatic System Reflex Points: The webbing between the fingers indicates the lymphatic system. Gently massaging these regions can improve lymphatic drainage, boost immunological function, and reduce edema.

Shoulder and Arm Reflex Points: The outside border of the palm, extending from the base of the little finger to the wrist, corresponds to the shoulders and arms. Stimulating this region can help alleviate shoulder stress and arm stiffness.

Hip and Leg Reflex Points: The base of the palm, near the wrist, represents the hips and legs. Massaging this region can aid with hip pain, sciatica, and leg discomfort.

Solar Plexus: The solar plexus reflex point is situated in the center of the palm, right beneath the middle finger. Stimulating this area can aid with stress reduction, relaxation, and overall well-being.

How Does Reflexology Work?

Reflexology is a holistic therapy based on the principle that specific points on the hands, feet and ears correspond to different parts of the body. By applying pressure to these reflex sites, you strive to promote healing, alleviate tension and restore equilibrium within the body. Here, we look into the processes of reflexology and how it works.

Reflex Points and Corresponding Body Parts:

Reflexology organizes the hands and feet into reflex zones, each correlating to distinct organs, glands and systems. For example, the tips of the fingers and toes correspond to the head and brain and the arch of the foot corresponds to the spine. By stimulating these locations, you can alter the associated bodily areas, improving a healthy lifestyle.

Nerve Pathway and Energy Flow:

One explanation for reflexology is that it operates via neural pathways. The body comprises a complicated network of nerves that connects the brain to other organs and tissues.

Reflex points are hypothesized to function as mini-gateways, with pressure sending messages across these neural pathways and eliciting a reaction in the surrounding region.

Traditional Chinese medicine offers another perspective, viewing the body as a linked system of energy channels known as **meridians**. Reflex points are identified as nodes on these meridians. Stimulating them promotes energy flow Qi (), restoring balance and harmony to the body.

Circulatory and Lymphatic System Stimulation:

Reflexology can also enhance blood and lymphatic circulation. Applying pressure on reflex points can increase blood flow to certain organs, improving oxygen and nutrient delivery while also assisting in the elimination of toxins and waste items. Improved circulation promotes general health and speeds up the healing process.

Reflexology is also beneficial to the lymphatic system, which is important for immunological function and fluid balance. By activating lymphatic drainage reflex sites, practitioners can improve the body's ability to cleanse and fight infections, hence strengthening the immune system.

Stress Reduction and Relaxation:

One of the most obvious advantages of reflexology is its ability to alleviate tension and induce relaxation. Stress may have a harmful influence on many physiological systems, causing a variety of health problems. Reflexology activates the body's relaxation response, which reduces tension and lowers stress chemicals like cortisol.

During a reflexology treatment, the parasympathetic nervous system (which controls relaxation and digestion) is triggered. This causes a drop in heart rate, blood pressure, and muscular tension, resulting in a state of profound relaxation. Regular sessions can assist with chronic stress, sleep quality, and general well-being.

Pain Relief with Endorphin Release:

Reflexology is well-recognized for its pain-relieving properties. Applying pressure on reflex sites might cause the release of endorphins, the body's natural pain relievers. Endorphins not only relieve pain but also increase feelings of well-being and joy.

This pain-relieving process makes reflexology useful for headaches, migraines, arthritis, and chronic pain. Practitioners can help people suffering from these diseases by focusing on certain reflex spots.

Balancing Body Systems:

Reflexology supports homeostasis, or the body's ability to maintain internal equilibrium in the face of external change. Reflexology regulates a variety of physiological systems, including the digestive, endocrine, respiratory, and circulatory.

For example, activating the digestive system's reflex points can improve digestion, reduce bloating, and alleviate constipation. Similarly, focusing on the endocrine system's reflex points can aid in hormone balance, treating conditions like thyroid abnormalities and adrenal exhaustion. Reflexology promotes general health and well-being by supporting the body's inherent regulating processes.

Scientific Research and Theories:

While reflexology has a long history of usage throughout cultures, scientific study into its mechanics and efficacy is still underway. Some studies have yielded encouraging benefits, notably in terms of stress reduction, pain alleviation, and better quality of life for individuals with chronic diseases.

Tension Reduction: Several studies have found that reflexology may greatly reduce tension and anxiety. For example, research published in the journal Complementary Therapies in Clinical Practice discovered that patients who had reflexology reported decreased stress and improved happiness.

Pain Relief: A study published in Pain Management Nursing found that reflexology can help cancer patients reduce pain and improve their quality of life. Another research published in The Journal of Nursing Research discovered that reflexology might help women with their menstrual discomfort.

Circulation Improvement: According to research published in The Journal of Alternative and Complementary Medicine, reflexology can enhance blood flow and oxygenation in the foot, indicating potential advantages for circulatory health.

Practical Application in Reflexology

To properly utilize reflexology, practitioners must first understand how it works. Here's a step-by-step tutorial for doing a simple reflexology session on the hand.

Preparation: Create a peaceful and comfortable setting. The customer should be comfortable, whether sitting or lying down. Wash and warm your hands before beginning the workout.

Warm-up: Start with mild hand massages to relax the client's hands and increase blood flow. Use circular motions for the palms and mild strokes for the fingers.

Identify Reflex Points: Use a reflexology chart to find major reflex points on your hands. Familiarize yourself with the postures and their respective body components.

Pressure: Using your thumb and fingers, gently yet firmly press each reflex point. Use techniques like thumb walking, which involves pressing and moving your thumb in little increments along the reflex zones.

Observation: Pay attention to how the customer responds. Sensitivity in certain regions may signal imbalances or difficulties in the corresponding bodily components. Adjust your pressure to guarantee comfort.

Concentrate on Problem Areas: Spend more attention on reflex points that correspond to the client's unique health issues. For example, if they have digestion problems, concentrate on the middle palm area.
Close the session with mild hand massages to help the client relax and conclude the therapy. Encourage them to drink water afterward to help eliminate toxins.

Reflexology works by stimulating the nerves, improving circulation, reducing tension, and providing pain relief. Practitioners who understand the body's reflex spots and the mechanics underlying reflexology can successfully promote healing and harmony inside the body. While more study is needed to completely understand its mechanics, existing data and centuries of practice back up reflexology's benefits as a holistic therapy.1

CHAPTER 3

HAND REFLEXOLOGY PREPARATIONS AND PRECAUTIONS

Contraindications and Safety Considerations:

Hand reflexology, like any other therapeutic technique, has its own set of contraindications and safety precautions that must be followed to protect the client's well-being. Understanding these factors is critical for any practitioner who wishes to provide safe and effective therapies.

1. Medical conditions and contraindications:

Certain medical issues necessitate caution or may even be inappropriate for hand reflexology. These include serious circulation issues such as deep vein thrombosis, severe varicose veins, and uncontrolled high blood pressure. Reflexology may also be ineffective for those who have serious illnesses, recent operations, or hand fractures. Autoimmune disorders and severe inflammatory problems may need a more careful approach, requiring the practitioner to collaborate closely with the client's healthcare physician.

2. Pregnancy:

While reflexology can be useful during pregnancy, it should be used with caution, particularly during the first trimester. Reflex points considered to affect the reproductive system should be avoided. Always speak with the client's healthcare physician before starting.

3. Skin conditions:

Reflexology can worsen skin disorders including eczema, psoriasis, and open sores on the hands. In such circumstances, avoid direct contact with the afflicted regions and use gentle measures to minimize discomfort or additional aggravation.

4. Psychological conditions:

For clients with significant mental health difficulties, particularly those involving trauma or extreme anxiety, it is critical that reflexology treatments do not unwittingly elicit unpleasant emotions. Creating a secure and supportive atmosphere is essential.

5. **Allergies and sensitivities:**

Some customers may be allergic to certain oils, lotions, or sanitizing agents used during reflexology. Always inquire about any known allergies or sensitivities before commencing a session, and use hypoallergenic materials as needed.

6. **Communicating with clients:**

Clear communication with customers about their medical history and any concerns they may have is essential. A good intake form can assist collect the relevant information. Furthermore, practitioners should describe the scope and limitations of reflexology, emphasizing that it is a supplementary therapy rather than a replacement for medical treatment.

7. **Modifying Techniques:**

Techniques must be adjusted to meet the demands of each individual customer. Gentler procedures may be required for older customers or those with fragile hands. Similarly, with youngsters, less pressure should be used and sessions should be shorter.

8. **Emergency protocols:**

Practitioners should be prepared for any potential emergency by establishing a clear protocol. This involves being able to identify indicators of discomfort or bad reactions and having emergency contact information readily available.

9. **Professional Boundaries:**

Maintaining professional boundaries is vital for creating a safe and courteous atmosphere. This involves respecting the client's degree of comfort with touch and always obtaining consent before initiating therapy.

Finally, it is critical to recognize and follow contraindications and safety precautions when doing hand reflexology. This protects both the client's safety and comfort, as well as the practitioner's reputation and professionalism. By focusing on these elements, reflexologists may provide treatments that are both effective and reassuring, building trust and beneficial outcomes for their clients.

Preparing Yourself and The Client

An effective hand reflexology treatment requires thorough preparation. Both the practitioner and the client must be well prepared to guarantee a happy and therapeutic encounter. Here, we'll look at the important stages for preparing yourself and your client for a reflexology session.

1. **Prepare Yourself:**
As a reflexologist, your physical and mental condition have a big impact on the quality of the session. Begin by ensuring that you are well-rested and free of any physical discomfort that may impair your ability to perform skills efficiently. Mental preparation is also vital; practice activities that encourage tranquility and

attention, such as meditation, deep breathing exercises, or a short stroll.

2. **Personal Hygiene:**

Maintaining good levels of personal cleanliness is essential. Make sure your hands are clean and free of unpleasant scents. Nails should be clipped and smoothed to avoid scratching the client's skin. Wear little or no jewelry to reduce pain or distractions during the session.

3. **Professional appearance:**

Dress in comfortable, professional apparel that allows you ease of movement while maintaining a neat look. This promotes a professional atmosphere and instills confidence in your customers.

4. **Mental preparation:**

Mental preparation is freeing your thoughts of distractions and concentrating on the impending session. Establish a conscious presence, which helps you to completely focus on the client's demands. This may be accomplished by engaging in a brief meditation session or simply taking a few minutes to focus on oneself.

5. **Preparing the Client:**

Before the appointment, discuss explicitly with the client about what they may expect. Provide information on the advantages of hand reflexology, the techniques that will be utilized, and any feelings they may feel. Encourage the customer to ask questions and share any concerns they may have.

6. **Health Intake Form:**

Have the client fill out a detailed health intake form. This should include medical history, current health problems, allergies, and any specific topics they want to discuss during the session. Reviewing this information enables you to personalize the program to their unique requirements while avoiding any contraindications.

7. **Client's Comfort:**

Ensure that the customer is comfortable during the session. This begins with providing a friendly and relaxing atmosphere. Offer them a nice seat or reclining chair where they may unwind. Provide support cushions as needed, and keep the room temperature reasonable.

8. **Emotional Preparedness:**

Address any emotional issues that the client may have. Some clients may be nervous about starting a new therapy or experiencing physical contact. Take the time to comfort them, explain the procedure in detail, and encourage them to talk freely during the session.

9. **Informed consent:**

Obtain the client's informed permission before commencing the session. This includes discussing the nature of reflexology, its advantages, and any potential hazards. Ensure that the client understands and agrees with the treatment strategy.

10. **Grounding Techniques:**

Before beginning, practice grounding skills with the client. This may involve deep breathing exercises or a brief guided meditation. Grounding allows both the client and practitioner to become completely present, resulting in a more productive and connected session.

11. **Hydration & Comfort:**

Encourage the client to drink water before and following the session. Hydration aids the detoxifying process and improves the efficiency of reflexology. Ensure that they are comfortable in their attire and position during the session.

In conclusion, significant preparation by both the practitioner and the client is required for a successful hand reflexology session. By addressing physical, mental, and emotional preparedness, as well as assuring clear communication and comfort, you may create a healing and relaxing atmosphere. This comprehensive approach not only improves therapeutic outcomes but also fosters trust and connection with your clients, resulting in a more satisfying reflexology practice.

Setting Up the Treatment Space

A relaxing and professional treatment environment is crucial for a successful hand reflexology session. The setting has a huge impact on the client's relaxation and overall experience. Here's a thorough guide on creating the optimal treatment area.

1. **Location:**

Choose a peaceful, accessible spot for your treatment area. Whether it's a dedicated room in your house, a professional clinic, or a transportable setup, the environment should be quiet and distraction-free. Privacy is critical in making clients feel comfortable and safe.

2. **Ambiance:**

The therapy room's environment is important in encouraging relaxation. Aim for a relaxing and friendly environment. Soft illumination, such as dimmable lights or candles, may have a relaxing effect. Natural light is useful, but it should be controlled to prevent glare.

3. **Decor and colours:**

Choose décor and colors that promote relaxation. Soft, neutral colors such as beige, mild blues, and greens are suitable. Avoid using extremely bright or vivid hues, which may be stimulating. Simple, attractive design, such as plants, delicate artwork, and minimalist furniture, contributes to the relaxing atmosphere.

4. **Aromatherapy:**

Aromatherapy can help you relax more. Essential oils such as lavender, chamomile, and eucalyptus can be diffused to generate a relaxing scent. Make sure the fragrances are subtle and not overpowering since strong odors can be distracting or uncomfortable for certain customers.

5. **Furniture & Layout:**

Comfortable sitting is crucial. A reclining chair or massage table with customizable settings enables clients to select the most comfortable position. Ensure that the back and arms are well supported. Arrange furniture to allow for easy mobility around the client, allowing the practitioner can operate successfully without strain.

6. Cleaning and Hygiene:

Maintain a high level of cleanliness throughout the treatment area. Clean your floors, surfaces, and equipment regularly. Use fresh linens for each customer and sterilize all instruments. A clutter-free atmosphere promotes a sense of tranquility and professionalism.

7. Temperature Control:

Ensure that the room temperature is comfortable. Too hot or too chilly temperatures might impair the client's ability to relax. If necessary, provide blankets or heating pads, and keep the room ventilated to avoid drafts.

8. **Sound and music:**

Soft, peaceful music or natural noises might improve the relaxation experience. Keep the volume low enough to be calming but not distracting. Avoid music with lyrics or sudden changes in pace. White noise devices can also aid in hiding extraneous sounds.

9. **Essential supplies:**

Keep all of your supplies within easy reach. This includes lotions or oils, towels, hand sanitizers, and any reflexology instruments you might use. A small table or cart can help you organize these goods more efficiently. Ensure that any items utilized are hypoallergenic and appropriate for the client's needs.

10. **Personal touches:**

Adding personal touches might improve the client's comfort. A simple water station with infused water, herbal teas, or a dish of fresh fruit will help clients feel welcome. Offering a warm cloth or a gentle hand massage as part of the preparation might be a nice touch.

11. **Professional Boundaries:** Establish clear professional boundaries in the environment. This includes establishing a separate room for consultations and intake paperwork, so that confidential information may be handled privately. A clear separation between the treatment room and the rest of the space promotes a professional atmosphere.

12. Implement safety steps to create a secure atmosphere. This involves keeping a first-aid kit on hand, knowing where the emergency exits are, and ensuring that the treatment space is safe. Regularly inspect and resolve any possible safety hazards.

13. **Accessibility:** Make the treatment area accessible to all patients, including those with impairments. Make sure there are no impediments to mobility and that seating is easily available. If feasible, provide adaptable equipment to meet a variety of physical demands.

14. Consider incorporating digital conveniences for a contemporary touch. This might include a tablet or computer for booking appointments, viewing client data, or practicing guided meditation. Ensure that all digital gadgets are utilized discreetly and do not disturb the peaceful environment.

15. Refreshment Area: If space allows, set up a modest refreshment area where customers may unwind before or after their sessions. Offer water, herbal teas, and nutritious snacks. Clients can also use this section to fill out intake forms or read reflexology literature.

16. **Reflecting Space:** A modest reflecting room with comfortable chairs and motivational reading materials can help customers gather their thoughts and relax before or after their session. This can improve the whole therapeutic experience and offer value to your services.

To summarize, developing an optimal treatment area for hand reflexology requires great attention to detail as well as a focus on providing a calm, professional, and friendly environment. Consider ambiance, comfort, cleanliness, and accessibility to ensure that both you and your clients feel calm and supported. This comprehensive approach not only improves treatment efficacy but also develops trust and pleasant relationships with your clients, resulting in a more successful reflexology practice.

Hygiene and Sanitation

Hand reflexology requires rigorous cleanliness and sanitation standards to ensure the safety and well-being of both the practitioner and the client. Cleanliness promotes a professional workplace, reduces the transmission of illnesses, and improves the overall therapeutic experience. This is a complete guide to developing appropriate hygiene and sanitation practices.

1. **Personal Hygiene:** As a reflexologist, you must maintain proper personal hygiene. Begin with clean hands; thoroughly cleanse them with soap and water before and after each session. Use a nail brush to clean under your nails, where germs can collect. Maintain short, smooth nails to prevent scratching the client's skin. Avoid wearing strong fragrances or colognes, since they may be overwhelming and distracting.

2. Hand sanitization is a necessary procedure before touching the customer. Use an alcohol-based hand sanitizer containing at least 60% alcohol. This guarantees that any remaining germs are eliminated. It is also a good idea to sanitize your hands in front of the customer to demonstrate your devotion to hygiene.

3. **Equipment Sterilization:** All tools and equipment used during the session must be sanitized both before and after usage. This contains all reflexology instruments, such as rollers and massage sticks. Cleaning these products using medical-grade disinfectants and

following the manufacturer's recommendations will ensure proper sterilization. For goods that cannot be sanitized, consider using disposable options.

4. **Linens and Towels:** Each client should receive new linens, towels, and any other cloth materials used during the session. To kill germs and bacteria, wash these items in hot water with the appropriate detergent. Use hypoallergenic detergents to avoid skin reactions. Clean linens should be stored in a closed cabinet to avoid dust and contamination.

5. **Treatment Area Cleanliness:** The treatment area should be cleaned and sanitized regularly. This includes wiping down surfaces with disinfectant wipes, mopping the floors with an appropriate cleaner, and regularly sanitizing all high-touch areas (such as doorknobs and light switches). To keep the room's air clean, use air purifiers with HEPA filters.

6. **Waste Management:** Effective waste management is essential. Place any single-use items, such as gloves or tissues, in a lined trash can with a lid. To avoid odors and bacterial growth, empty and sanitize your trash can regularly. Follow local regulations when disposing of medical or hazardous waste.

7. **Glove Use:** Wearing gloves may be required in some cases, particularly if the client's hands have open wounds or skin conditions. Use disposable gloves and replace them between clients. Make sure you are not allergic to latex gloves; if you are, use nitrile or vinyl alternatives.

8. **Sanitizing Products:** Choose sanitizing products that are effective yet gentle on the skin. Alcohol-based sanitizers, disinfectant wipes, and antimicrobial soaps are good options. Ensure that these products are readily available and used consistently. Consider using hypoallergenic and fragrance-free products to prevent any adverse reactions.

9. **Educating customers:** Educate your customers on the significance of hygiene and sanitation in reflexology. Inform them about your practices and advise them to wash their hands before the session. Providing hand sanitizer for clients to use upon arrival might also be advantageous.

10. **Practitioner Wellness:** Your health and wellness are crucial. If you are feeling poorly, it's advisable to reschedule sessions to minimize spreading illness. Regularly monitor your health and be alert to any signs. Staying hydrated, eating a balanced diet, and getting appropriate rest are vital for supporting your immune system and general well-being.

11. **Continual Monitoring:** Regularly examine and update your hygiene and sanitation procedures. Stay informed about new guidelines and recommendations from health authorities. Conduct frequent reviews of your treatment area and equipment to verify they satisfy cleanliness

requirements. Implement input from clients to enhance your methods consistently.

12. **Professional Cleaners:** Consider hiring professional cleaners for deep cleaning jobs. This ensures that areas beyond your daily routine, such as carpets, upholstery, and hard-to-reach spots, are thoroughly cleaned. Schedule extensive cleaning sessions periodically to maintain a perfect atmosphere.

In conclusion, strict cleanliness and sanitation standards are important to the success of a hand reflexology practice. By emphasizing cleanliness, you not only preserve the health of your clients and yourself but also boost the professionalism and integrity of your service. A clean and sanitary setting stimulates relaxation and healing, contributing to a happy and successful reflexology experience.

CHAPTER 4

HAND REFLEXOLOGY TECHNIQUES

In the complex realm of hand reflexology, the methods used are as varied as they are effective. From the fundamentals of thumb walking and finger walking to the more advanced techniques of rotations and hooking, each technique has a distinct function in promoting health and well-being. This chapter digs thoroughly into the foundational principles of hand reflexology, providing both new and seasoned practitioners with a complete guide to mastering this ancient discipline. Furthermore, the integration of tools and assistance will be investigated, emphasizing how these instruments may improve accuracy and efficacy.

Basic techniques:

Basic techniques include thumb walking, finger walking, and pressure techniques.

Hand reflexology starts with a thorough grasp of the fundamental methods. These strategies serve as the foundation for every practitioner's ability to provide successful and therapeutic therapies.

Thumb walking is one of the most basic methods in hand reflexology. This procedure entails applying consistent, rhythmic pressure to the hand's reflex zones using the thumb. The action mimics that of a caterpillar, with the thumb bending and straightening as it moves over the skin. This method is very good for covering large portions of the palm and may be done with varied degrees of pressure to accommodate the client's comfort level. Thumb walking not only stimulates reflex spots, but it also improves circulation, decreases tension, and promotes relaxation all across the body.

Finger walking is a supplementary method that uses the fingers, usually the index or middle finger, to travel smaller or more sensitive portions of the hand. This approach is useful for identifying particular reflex spots, such as those on the fingers or around the knuckle. By altering the pressure and tempo, practitioners may personalize finger walking to each client's specific requirements. This approach is very useful for targeting certain regions that may need further attention since it provides a better degree of precision and control.

The interaction of thumb walking and finger walking provides a thorough approach to hand reflexology. Finger walking allows for more precise therapy on individual reflex sites, while thumb walking covers wider regions and gives overall treatment. Together, these strategies provide a balanced and efficient manner of activating the whole hand.

Pressure techniques are another important aspect of hand reflexology. This approach includes applying direct, persistent pressure to a reflex spot using the thumb or fingers. By applying pressure to a particular location, practitioners may relieve stress, increase blood flow, and stimulate the associated organ or body component. Pressure methods are very effective for treating chronic pain, intestinal difficulties, and other persistent diseases. This procedure requires a thorough awareness of the hand's response zones, as well as a delicate touch, to ensure that the pressure delivered is therapeutic rather than painful.

Each of these fundamental methods is essential to the practice of hand reflexology. By learning thumb walking, finger walking, and pressure methods, practitioners may provide treatments that are both thorough and precise, addressing each client's specific requirements.

Advanced techniques:

Advanced techniques include rotations, hooking, and point pressing. Building based on fundamental procedures, advanced approaches such as rotations, hooking, and point pressing enable practitioners to go further into hand reflexology's therapeutic advantages. These approaches provide more specific and intense treatments, making them useful for experienced practitioners.

Rotations are performed by moving the thumb or fingers in tiny, circular movements over a reflex point. This approach helps to relieve congestion, increase energy flow, and promote healing in certain locations. Rotations may be done at various pressure levels, enabling practitioners to tailor the method to the client's demands. This therapy is very useful for treating tight or knotted regions, offering a subtle but strong kind of relaxation. Rotations may provide great alleviation and generate a feeling of well-being for clients suffering from muscle tension or stress.

Hooking is a specific method in which the thumb or finger is used to **hook** onto a reflex point and then gently draw it out. This movement alleviates deep-seated stress and provides a profound sensation of relaxation. Hooking is especially useful on the sides of the fingers and around the joints, where stress often develops. This method takes expertise and sensitivity since it entails delivering exact pressure to tiny places while avoiding pain. Hooking, when done properly, may considerably improve the therapeutic benefits of a reflexology session, making it an effective technique for treating chronic pain and stress.

Point pressing is the process of exerting hard, direct pressure on a particular reflex point over a prolonged period. This approach is quite successful in promoting healing and relieving pain in specific places. Point pressing requires a thorough understanding of the hand's reflex map, since practitioners must precisely target the spots corresponding to the client's complaints. This approach is very effective for treating acute conditions including headaches, nasal difficulties, and localized discomfort. By applying continuous pressure to the right reflex sites, practitioners may stimulate the body's natural healing processes and give considerable comfort to clients.

The use of these approaches enable practitioners to provide more nuanced and effective therapies. Rotations, hooking, and point pressing all have distinct advantages, and when coupled with fundamental methods, they provide a complete approach to hand reflexology that may treat a broad variety of health conditions.

Using Tools And Aids

Hand reflexology treatments can be substantially more precise and successful when instruments and assistance are used. Tools like **reflexology sticks, rollers,** and **acupressure rings** provide practitioners with greater alternatives for applying pressure and activating reflex sites, minimizing strain on their hands and allowing for more extensive sessions.

Reflexology sticks, usually made of wood or crystal, are used to apply precise pressure with ease. These sticks are great for working on tiny, precise points or locations that are tough to access with only the fingers. Practitioners may use a reflexology stick to apply pressure without becoming fatigued, allowing them to conduct longer sessions. These instruments also provide more control over the amount of pressure used, ensuring that treatments are both effective and pleasant for clients.

Rollers are other tools that can be used to massage larger portions of the hand, creating a pleasant, rolling pressure that improves relaxation and circulation. These instruments are especially useful for warming up the hands at the start of a session or giving a mild, all-over massage at the finish. Rollers come in a variety of sizes and materials, enabling practitioners to choose the one that best meets their requirements and those of their clients.

Acupressure rings are composed of coiled metal and may be rolled up and down the fingers to stimulate many reflex sites at once. These rings are great for improving circulation, easing stress, and offering a unique sensory experience. They may be included in a routine or provided to clients as a form of self-care in between sessions. Acupressure rings are simple to use and may be integrated into any reflexology session to provide an additional layer of stimulation and relaxation.

The use of instruments and assistance in hand reflexology provides various advantages. These tools may improve treatment accuracy, minimize hand strain for practitioners, and give clients a more diverse and pleasurable experience. Practitioners may improve their technique by using equipment like reflexology sticks, rollers, and acupressure rings to provide more effective and thorough treatments.

In conclusion, hand reflexology demands a solid grasp of both fundamental and advanced methods. Thumb walking, finger walking, and pressure methods provide the basis for successful treatments, whilst rotations, hooking, and point pressing provide deeper, more specific therapeutic alternatives. Incorporating tools and assistance improves the accuracy and efficacy of treatments, making hand reflexology a diverse and powerful technique for improving health and wellness.

Practitioners may realize the full potential of hand reflexology by refining their abilities and experimenting with new methods. This ancient technique takes a comprehensive approach to healing, addressing the body's physical, mental, and energy requirements. Practitioners may deliver thorough and successful treatments that promote balance, relaxation, and general well-being by integrating basic approaches with advanced practices as well as tools and assistance.

CHAPTER 5

REFLEX ZONES OF THE HAND

Hand reflexology is based on the idea that certain portions of the hand connect to various sections of the body. This detailed map of reflex zones serves as the foundation for therapeutic approaches designed to improve general health and well-being. Anyone wishing to learn hand reflexology must first understand the philosophy underlying zone treatment, as well as precise maps of hand reflex zones and reflex sites for each bodily system.

Zone Therapy Theory

The notion of zone treatment stretches back to ancient cultures, but it was codified in the early twentieth century by Dr. William H. Fitzgerald and expanded upon by Eunice Ingham. According to zone treatment, the body may be divided into 10 longitudinal zones, which extend from the top of the head to the tips of the toes and fingers. Each zone relates to a distinct organ or bodily component.

Hand reflexology involves mirroring these zones on the hands, with each finger representing a vertical slice of the body. For example, the thumb belongs to the head and neck, but the little finger is associated with the body's extremities. This theoretical framework lays forth a strategy for finding and treating reflex sites on the hands that may affect comparable body regions.

The zone treatment hypothesis is based on the concept that energy flows across these zones. Disrupting this energy flow might cause pain or sickness. By applying pressure to the reflex points within these zones, reflexologists hope to restore balance and harmony while also stimulating the body's natural healing processes.

Detailed maps of hand reflex zones

A thorough map of the hand reflex zones is required for successful hand reflexology. These maps show the particular locations of reflex sites for numerous organs, glands, and body parts. Understanding these maps enables reflexologists to tailor their therapies accurately.

The thumb is mostly related to the head and neck area. Reflex points on the thumb may be utilized to treat disorders with the brain, sinuses, pituitary gland, and thyroid gland. For example, the tip of the thumb correlates to the brain, making it an ideal target for headaches or mental tiredness.

The fingers symbolize various areas of the body. The index finger connects to the upper body, which includes the eyes, ears, and neck. The middle finger belongs to the chest and upper back, and the ring finger is related to the abdomen. The little finger symbolizes the lower body, which includes the legs and feet.

The Palm: The palm is split into various zones, each representing a major organ or bodily system. The center portion of the palm relates to the stomach, liver, and pancreas, while the area below the little finger refers to the heart and lungs. The reproductive organs and lower abdomen are connected with the palm's base, near the wrist.

The Back of the Hand: Although less typically utilized, the back of the hand does include reflex points. These spots may help with spinal and nervous system disorders. The region between the knuckles correlates to the spinal column, and concentrating on these areas may assist with back discomfort and posture.

The Hand's Sides: The extremities of the body are represented by the hand's exterior borders, including the sides of the fingers. These locations are important for resolving difficulties with the arms, legs, and joints. For example, the region along the hand's outside border, from the base of the little finger to the wrist, is connected to the hip and leg.

Detailed maps of these zones let practitioners traverse the complicated environment of the hand with confidence. By referring to these maps, reflexologists may guarantee that they are applying pressure to the precise places to obtain the intended therapeutic results.

Understanding Reflex Points for Each Body System

Effective hand reflexology requires a thorough awareness of each bodily system's reflex sites. This understanding helps practitioners to personalize their therapies to individual health conditions while promoting general well-being.

The Nervous System: Reflex sites for the nervous system are typically found on the fingers and the center of the palm. The tips of the fingers connect to the brain, whereas the region surrounding the base of the thumb is associated with the spinal cord. Working on these issues may assist in reducing stress, anxiety, and neurological diseases.

The respiratory system's reflex points are located on the thumb and the region below the little finger. The tip of the thumb connects to the nose and sinuses, whereas the region below the little finger is associated with the lungs and bronchial tubes. These principles may help cure respiratory problems including asthma, bronchitis, and allergies.

The Digestive System: The digestive system is shown on the palm. The palm's center section relates to the stomach, liver, and pancreas, while the area under the index and middle fingers refers to the intestines. Applying pressure to these sites helps alleviate digestive problems such as indigestion, constipation, and irritable bowel syndrome.

The circulatory system's reflex points are located below the little finger and at the base of the thumb. The region under the little finger relates to the heart, whereas the base of the thumb connects to the arteries and veins. Working on these principles may enhance blood circulation and reduce cardiovascular diseases.

The endocrine system, which contains glands that create hormones, is shown on the fingers and the center of the palm. The pituitary and pineal glands are located at the ends of the fingers, whereas the thyroid gland is located around the base of the thumb. These points are useful for hormone imbalances and metabolic problems.

The musculoskeletal system's reflex points are located on the back of the hand and the sides of the fingers. The space between the knuckles connects to the spine, whereas the sides of the fingers connect to the arms, legs, and joints. Applying pressure to these sites helps alleviate musculoskeletal problems such as arthritis, muscular discomfort, and joint stiffness.

The reproductive system is shown on the base of the palm, close to the wrist. This region corresponds to the ovaries, testes, and other reproductive organs. Working on these topics may assist with reproductive health difficulties including menstruation discomfort, infertility, and prostate disorders.

Reflexologists can deliver focused therapies that address particular health conditions since they understand the reflex regions for each bodily system. This understanding enables them to design personalized reflexology treatments that promote balance and healing throughout the body.

Effective hand reflexology requires mastery of the hand's reflex zones. Zone therapy theory offers a framework for comprehending how various locations of the body are linked via reflex sites on the hands. Detailed maps of hand reflex zones provide a visual aid for finding these locations, whilst a thorough grasp of reflex points for each bodily system allows practitioners to personalize their therapies to particular health conditions.

Putting this information into practice, helps reflexologists provide effective and holistic therapies that improve general health and well-being. Hand reflexology provides a varied and successful method of healing, both for chronic diseases, relieving stress and improving overall well-being.

CHAPTER 6

HAND REFLEXOLOGY FOR COMMON AILMENTS

Hand reflexology provides a non-invasive, holistic way of treating a variety of common diseases. By stimulating certain reflex sites on the hands, practitioners may promote healing, alleviate symptoms and improve general health. Here are how hand reflexology can be used to treat headaches and migraines, stress and anxieties, digestive disorders, respiratory problems, muscles pain, joint pain and general health problems.

Headaches and Migraines:

Headaches and migraines are frequent conditions that may have a substantial influence on one's everyday life. Hand reflexology is a natural method for relieving the pain and suffering associated with these diseases. The reflex points on the hands that correlate to the head, neck, and brain are very beneficial for relieving headaches and migraines.

Start by concentrating on the thumb, which depicts the head and neck. To treat the neck reflex point, push on the base of the thumb, since stress in the neck may frequently lead to headaches. Next, move your thumb down to its length, giving careful attention to the pad that represents the brain and pituitary gland. This method assists in relieving stress and promotes circulation in the head and neck area.

Furthermore, the tips of the fingers correspond to the head and can be used to treat headache symptoms. Finger strolling over the length of each finger, beginning at the base and progressing to the tip. This procedure stimulates the reflex spots on the skull, which promotes relaxation and pain alleviation. Combining these techniques can help reduce the frequency and severity of headaches and migraines, offering a natural and holistic solution.

Stress & Anxiety:

Stress and anxiety are common problems that may harm both mental and physical health. Hand reflexology provides a calming and therapeutic approach to treating these conditions. You will alleviate tension and promote relaxation by focusing on reflex points related to the neurological system and adrenal glands.

Begin by concentrating on the solar plexus reflex point in the middle of the palm. Apply gentle pressure with thumb walking or point pressing techniques. The solar plexus is a major nerve center that can help to relax the nervous system and reduce stress. Encourage the client to take calm, deep breaths while you focus on this spot to maximize the relaxing impact.

Next, proceed to the adrenal gland reflex points, which are located at the base of the thumbs. To stimulate these points, stroll with your thumbs or press them. The adrenal glands create hormones that control stress and stimulating these reflex regions assists in balancing hormone levels and ease anxiety.

Practicing mindfulness and deep breathing techniques throughout the reflexology session might further improve the effects. Encourage the client to concentrate on their breath and be present, which may help to calm the mind and eliminate nervous thoughts. By treating both the physical and emotional components of stress and anxiety, hand reflexology offers a complete approach to enhancing mental health.

Digestive Issues:

Digestive disorders, such as bloating, constipation, and indigestion, may cause severe pain and damage overall health. Hand reflexology may assist in reducing these symptoms by activating reflex points involved with the digestive system, facilitating improved digestion and bowel motions.

Begin by concentrating on the palm, where the reflex points for the stomach, intestines, and liver are situated. To enhance digestive health, stimulate these regions by thumb walking while giving firm, constant pressure. Begin with the top portion of the palm, focusing on the stomach and liver reflex points. Move to the center of the palm, where the intestines' reflex points are located.

Next, concentrate on the wrists, which contain reflex points for the lower back and intestines. Use rotation and hooking methods to stimulate these spots, which will aid digestion and relieve constipation. Firm pressure on the wrist's inner and outer margins may also improve therapy efficacy.

Encourage the client to drink lots of water and eat a nutritious diet to improve digestive health. Combining hand reflexology with lifestyle modifications may give a comprehensive approach to addressing digestive disorders and increasing overall health.

Respiratory Problems:

Asthma, bronchitis, and nasal congestion are all examples of respiratory issues that may cause severe pain and interfere with everyday activities. Hand reflexology may assist in reducing these problems by activating reflex sites connected with the respiratory system, enabling improved breathing and lowering symptoms.

Begin by concentrating on the top half of the palm, which has reflex points for the lungs and bronchial tubes. To improve respiratory health, stimulate these regions with thumb walking and provide firm, constant pressure. Move to the fingertips, which correspond to the sinus and nasal cavities. Finger-walking down the length of each finger stimulates these reflex sites, which helps to relieve sinus congestion and enhance breathing.

Next, concentrate on the base of the thumb, which represents the neck and throat. Use point pressing to stimulate this region, which may help relieve bronchitis and throat inflammation. Combining these approaches may assist in reducing respiratory issues, offering a natural and holistic approach to healthier breathing.

Encourage the client to undertake deep breathing exercises during the reflexology session to maximize the effects. Deep breathing expands the lungs and improves oxygen flow, which promotes overall respiratory health. Hand reflexology addresses both the physical and behavioural elements of respiratory disorders, providing a complete approach to improve breathing and symptom reduction.

Muscle and Joint Pain

Muscular and joint discomfort may have a substantial influence on everyday activities and overall well-being. Hand reflexology is a natural and efficient approach to relieve pain and promote healing by activating reflex sites in the muscles and joints.

Begin by concentrating on the palm, which has reflex points for the muscles and joints. To enhance muscle and joint health, stimulate these regions with thumb walking while delivering firm, constant pressure. Begin with the top half of the palm, focusing on the reflex spots in the shoulders and upper back. Move to the center of the palm, where the reflex points for the lower back and hips are located.

Next, concentrate on the fingers, which correlate to various sections of the body, such as the shoulders, arms, and legs. Finger walking down the length of each finger stimulates these reflex sites, which helps relieve muscular and joint discomfort. Pay specific attention to any places that seem especially tight or uncomfortable, and use point-pressing methods to relieve tension and encourage healing.

Massage treatments and heat therapy may be used during a reflexology session to improve the results. Massaging the hands and using warm compresses may assist in relaxing muscles and promote circulation, promoting overall muscle and joint health. Hand reflexology addresses both the physical and lifestyle components of muscle and joint pain, providing a holistic approach to pain relief and rehabilitation.

Enhancing Overall Well-Being

Hand reflexology is not only useful in treating particular disorders, but it also improves general health. By activating reflex spots connected to the body's many systems, practitioners may promote balance, relaxation, and general wellness.

Start by concentrating on the solar plexus reflex point, which is situated in the middle of the palm. Apply mild pressure using thumb walking or point pressing methods. The solar plexus is a significant nerve area that may aid to regulate the nervous system and induce relaxation. Encourage the client to take calm, deep breaths while you focus on this spot to maximize the relaxing impact.

The adrenal gland reflex points are positioned on the base of the thumbs. To stimulate these points, stroll with your thumbs or press them. The adrenal glands create hormones that control stress, and stimulating these reflex sites may assist in balancing hormone levels and improve general health.

Concentrate on the digestive system's reflex spots in the center of the hand. Thumb walking stimulates these regions, which promotes improved digestion and general wellness. Move to the tips of your fingers, which correlate to the head and sinuses, and use finger walking to activate these reflex sites and improve mental clarity.

Incorporating mindfulness and meditation activities into the reflexology treatment might increase the effects. Encourage the client to concentrate on their breathing and be present, which may help to calm the mind and increase general well-being. Combining hand reflexology with lifestyle modifications, such as eating a balanced diet and exercising regularly, may give a comprehensive approach to improving overall health and wellness.

Hand reflexology provides a diverse and comprehensive approach to treating common diseases and improving general well-being. By stimulating certain reflex sites on the hands, practitioners may promote healing, alleviate symptoms, and enhance general health. It is a natural and efficient treatment for headaches and migraines, stress and anxiety, digestive disorders, respiratory problems, and muscle and joint discomfort. By combining reflexology with complementary treatments and lifestyle modifications, practitioners may provide a holistic approach to health and well-being, resulting in a transforming healing experience.

CHAPTER 8

SPECIAL CONSIDERATIONS IN HAND REFLEXOLOGY

Hand reflexology can be adjusted to the specific requirements of each client. Practitioners may deliver more effective and individualized therapies by knowing and addressing the unique needs of different age groups, pregnant women, athletes and people with chronic diseases.

Reflexology for several age groups: children, adults, and the elderly

Hand reflexology benefits people of all ages, from toddlers to the elderly, but the approach and methods should be tailored to each age group's unique requirements and sensitivities.

Children:

Hand reflexology may help children with a variety of conditions, including anxiety, stomach disorders, and sleep disruptions. However, since their bodies are more sensitive, the pressure used should be moderate and the sessions should be shorter. Begin with a short description of what will happen, using basic language to ensure their comfort and relaxation. Engage them by making the session enjoyable and participatory for example, tell a relaxing narrative or play quiet music in the background.

During the session, concentrate on reflex spots that may ease common kid diseases. For example, gently massage the solar plexus point to mitigate anxiety and promote relaxation. Finger reflex points may help with nasal congestion and headaches, both of which are frequent among youngsters. Always monitor the child's response and modify the pressure and duration appropriately. It is also critical to interact with the parents to identify any particular concerns or problems that need care.

Adults:

Adults often use hand reflexology to reduce stress, ease pain, and promote general well-being. Adults have a larger tolerance for pressure, therefore pressures may be harsher than those used on children. Begin by addressing the client's medical history and particular issues to adapt the session to their requirements.

Focus on the adrenal gland reflex points in the center of your hands to relieve tension. Firm pressure on these spots may assist manage stress and increase energy levels. For people suffering from digestive problems, focus on the stomach and intestinal reflex points in the hands. Headaches and migraines may be relieved by concentrating on the reflex points on the tips of the fingers, especially the thumb, which relate to the head and neck.

Use relaxation methods such as deep breathing and awareness to boost the therapeutic benefits. Encourage customers to concentrate on their breathing and be present throughout the session. This may enhance the effects of reflexology by providing a deeper level of relaxation and stress reduction.

Elderly:

Hand reflexology can equally be very useful to the elderly, improving circulation, relieving pain and increasing mobility. However, seniors' skin and tissues might be more sensitive, so apply moderate pressure and proceed with caution.

Begin with a comprehensive consultation to identify any underlying health issues, medicines and areas of concern. Concentrate on reflex points that may aid with typical concerns for the aged, including arthritis, joint discomfort and circulation problems. For example, activating the spine's reflex points on the sides of the thumb may help relieve back discomfort and enhance mobility.

Gentle rotations and gentle pressure on the wrist region help improve circulation, which is often an issue for older persons. Move slowly and deliberately to prevent inflicting discomfort or suffering. Use calming methods such as a warm hand bath before the session to relax the muscles and joints, making the reflexology treatment more effective and enjoyable.

Reflexology for Pregnant Women

Hand reflexology helps pregnant women with typical pregnancy-related symptoms including nausea, back discomfort, edema and stress. However, it is critical to approach reflexology with care and understand the unique demands and contraindications of pregnancy.

Before beginning the session, do a thorough assessment to determine the person's pregnancy stage and any unique concerns or problems.

Always avoid reflex regions that may activate the uterus, such as those related to the reproductive system. Concentrate instead on spots that promote relaxation and mitigate frequent pregnancy discomforts.

To relieve nausea and morning sickness, gently stimulate the stomach and solar plexus reflex points in the palm's middle. These points can assist in relieving nausea and promoting calm. To relieve back pain, focus on the reflex points for the spine and lower back, which are positioned along the sides of the thumb and wrist.

Swelling in the hands and feet is a common problem during pregnancy. Lightly massaging the kidney and lymphatic system reflex points, which are situated in the middle of the palms and around the wrist, can help minimize fluid retention and enhance circulation. Pregnant women are more sensitive to touch, so always use soft, soothing gestures and avoid exerting excessive pressure.

Stress and anxiety may be common throughout pregnancy. Use relaxation methods such as deep breathing exercises and mindfulness to assist the person to relax and decrease tension. Encourage the person to concentrate on their breathing and envision a serene, tranquil setting. This not only improves the reflexology therapy but also supports the general health of both the mother and the baby.

Reflexology For Athletes

Athletes often seek hand reflexology to improve performance, avoid injuries and speed up recovery. Because of the high demands put on their bodies, reflexology is a perfect addition to orthodox sports medicine.

Begin with a thorough consultation to learn about the athlete's training regimen, particular objectives and any current ailments or areas of concern. Concentrate on reflex areas that can increase flexibility, minimize muscular tension and boost overall performance.

Work on the muscle and joint reflex points, which are situated throughout the palm and fingers, to relieve muscular tension and discomfort. Firm, persistent pressure on these spots help in reducing muscle stiffness and increasing flexibility. The reflex points for the spine, which are placed on the sides of the thumb, also help with back discomfort and posture.

To improve circulation and speed up healing, concentrate on the cardiovascular and lymphatic reflex points in the palms and wrists. These areas enhance blood flow, decrease inflammation and aid in the elimination of metabolic waste products from the muscles.

Adopt dynamic methods like rotations and hooks to trigger deep reflex areas and improve treatment outcomes. Athletes often have a better tolerance for pressure, allowing for harder approaches to deliver deeper stimulation and relaxation. Encourage athletes to include regular hand reflexology treatments into their training schedules to retain peak performance and avoid injuries.

Reflexology for Chronic Conditions

Hand reflexology may be an effective therapeutic technique for those suffering from chronic diseases, reducing pain, enhancing quality of life, and boosting general health. Chronic illnesses including arthritis, diabetes, and fibromyalgia need a personalized strategy to guarantee successful and safe treatment.

Begin with a thorough interview to determine the client's medical history, current medicines, and particular symptoms. For arthritis patients, concentrate on the joint reflex points, which are situated throughout the fingers and palms. To prevent irritating or producing discomfort in the joints, use slow, soothing motions. Light rotations and finger walking exercises may assist in decreasing inflammation and increasing mobility.

Reflexology also aids patients with diabetes to improve circulation and control symptoms like neuropathy. To boost insulin production and control blood sugar levels, focus on the pancreatic reflex points in the palm's middle. The cardiovascular reflex points, which are positioned in the middle of the palms and around the wrists, can help to improve circulation and lower the risk of diabetic problems.

Fibromyalgia is defined by widespread pain and fatigue. Hand reflexology, which focuses on muscle reflex regions across the palm and fingers can bring great comfort. Use mild, constant pressure to minimize overstimulation and keep the client comfortable. Also incorporate relaxation methods such as deep breathing and awareness to improve the overall therapeutic impact and induce calm.

For all chronic diseases, it's critical to interact with the client and change the pressure and methods according to their input and comfort level. Regular reflexology treatments do help people with chronic illnesses manage their symptoms, enhance their quality of life and get continuing support.

In conclusion, hand reflexology is a dynamic and adaptable treatment that may be adjusted to the specific demands of various age groups, pregnant women, athletes and those with chronic diseases. Practitioners may deliver more effective and individualized therapies by recognizing and addressing the unique needs of each group. Children respond best to gentle treatments and shorter sessions, whilst adults benefit from harder pressures and relaxation techniques. The elderly need a careful approach with light pressure, while pregnant women benefit from avoiding specific reaction spots and concentrating on relaxation and alleviation from typical pregnancy symptoms. Dynamic methods may help athletes improve their performance and recuperation, while regular reflexology treatments can provide comfort and support for those suffering from chronic diseases. By understanding these distinct factors, practitioners may provide a transforming and therapeutic reflexology experience that is personalized to the specific requirements of each individual.

CHAPTER 9

COMBINING HAND REFLEXOLOGY WITH OTHER PRACTICES

Aromatherapy

Aromatherapy, or the therapeutic use of essential oils, may considerably improve the efficacy of a hand reflexology session. Essential oils are concentrated plant extracts that retain the inherent therapeutic characteristics of their source, providing benefits ranging from stress reduction to immunological support. When these oils are coupled with the tactile stimulation of reflexology, they may provide a profoundly calming and healing experience.

Using essential oils:

To begin incorporating aromatherapy into a hand reflexology session, choose essential oils that are appropriate for the individual's requirements and tastes. For example, lavender is well-known for its relaxing and stress-relieving effects, making it great for those who are worried or suffer sleeplessness. Chamomile, another calming oil, may assist to decrease anxiety and promote relaxation. Sandalwood provides a grounding effect, which is excellent for individuals seeking emotional equilibrium.

Mode of Application:

There are various excellent ways to use essential oils in reflexology sessions. One way is to diffuse the oils throughout the therapy room. Using an essential oil diffuser disperses fragrant molecules into the air, resulting in a relaxing and pleasant ambiance. Even before reflexology's physical touch is performed, the person starts to relax.

Another option is to apply the oils topically. This may be accomplished by diluting a few drops of essential oil in a carrier oil like jojoba, almond, or coconut. This combination may be applied directly to the person's hands and wrists. This not only helps the oils' medicinal compounds to permeate the skin, but it also improves the sensory experience by providing fragrant advantages. The practitioner might start the session by gently rubbing this oil combination into the client's palms to prepare the reflex spots for deeper treatment.

Creating custom blends:

Customizing essential oil mixes based on an individual's personal requirements might bring even more advantages. For example, a mix of lavender, chamomile, and sandalwood may be used to treat high levels of tension or anxiety. This combination promotes profound relaxation and emotional harmony. A combination of peppermint, eucalyptus, and lemon may be both refreshing and rejuvenating for those looking for a stimulating encounter. These oils assist to calm the mind, excite the senses, and improve lung function.

Aromatherapy may improve reflexology techniques:

The use of aromatherapy with hand reflexology goes beyond just applying oils or spreading them in air. The practitioner may improve various reflexology procedures by using oils that address specific health conditions. For example, while working on respiratory reflex points, oils like eucalyptus or peppermint might be quite beneficial. Their natural characteristics aid to open up airways and encourage better breathing, which improves the overall effectiveness of the reflexology therapy.

Scent and Memory

Aromatherapy's capacity to connect fragrance with memory and emotion is a significant but frequently ignored component. The olfactory system is intimately linked to the limbic system of the brain, which regulates emotion, behavior, and long-term memory. Using pleasant and relaxing fragrances during a reflexology treatment might help practitioners develop good connections for their clients. Over time, the mere aroma of these oils may elicit a relaxation response, enhancing the advantages of reflexology treatments and assisting the client in better managing stress and anxiety in their everyday lives.

Acupressure & Acupuncture

Acupressure and acupuncture, two important components of Traditional Chinese Medicine (TCM), may be effortlessly combined with hand reflexology to give a holistic approach to health and well-being. Both methods operate on the premise of stimulating certain places in the body to balance the flow of Qi (energy) and facilitate healing.

Understanding acupoints and reflex points:

Acupoints are precise areas on the body where energy routes known as meridians may be accessed in Traditional Chinese Medicine. These spots are utilized to alter the flow of energy and are said to correlate to different organs and biological functions. Reflexology follows a similar premise, with reflex spots on the hands and feet correlating to various sections of the body. The overlap between both systems enables a seamless combination of acupressure and reflexology.

Mode of Applying Acupressure:

During a hand reflexology session, the practitioner may improve the outcome by administering acupressure to specific areas on the hands. For example, the LI-4 point, which is placed between the thumb and index finger, is believed to reduce headaches and tension. The practitioner may enhance the therapeutic benefits of reflexology by applying consistent pressure to this spot throughout the session, providing tension reduction and increasing relaxation.

Another significant acupoint is PC-8, which is positioned in the middle of the palm. This point is related to soothing the mind and reducing anxiety. Infusing acupressure on PC-8 while working on heart and lung reflex points might result in a potent synergy, increasing the total efficacy of the therapy.

Integrating Acupuncture:

For acupuncturists, combining needle insertion with reflexology may deliver significant therapeutic effects. Acupuncture is the insertion of tiny needles into particular acupoints to facilitate energy flow and healing. This approach may be used in concert with reflexology to treat more serious health conditions.

During a reflexology treatment, acupuncture needles may be put into critical acupoints on the hands. For example, needles may be inserted into LI-4 and PC-8 as the practitioner applies reflexology to corresponding parts of the hand. The needles usually remain in place during the reflexology session, enabling the acupoints and reflex points to be stimulated simultaneously.

Combining acupressure, acupuncture, and reflexology:

The combination of acupressure, acupuncture, and reflexology provides a comprehensive approach to therapy that treats the body, mind, and spirit. This combination may be especially beneficial for chronic diseases and complicated health problems that need a multifaceted approach.

For example, a person suffering from chronic migraines may benefit from a combination therapy that combines acupressure on LI-4 as well as acupuncture on other pain relief and stress sites. Reflexology may then be performed to the hand regions associated with the head, neck, and nerve system. This holistic treatment addresses the underlying causes of migraines, providing relief from symptoms and increasing general well-being.

Energetic Synergy

The energy synergy formed by combining these methods may help the body's natural healing processes. Acupressure and acupuncture increase the flow of Qi, whilst reflexology improves circulation and relaxation. Together, they generate a condition of balance and harmony, allowing the body to repair itself. This holistic approach is especially useful for illnesses that affect numerous bodily systems, such as digestive issues, hormone imbalances, and chronic pain.

Case Studies:
Chronic Fatigue Syndrome

Consider a case study of someone suffering from chronic fatigue syndrome (CFS). This syndrome is characterized by acute exhaustion that does not improve with rest and may be worsened by physical or mental exertion. A combination of acupressure, acupuncture, and reflexology may be very useful.

Begin by applying acupressure to sites on the leg, such as ST-36 (Zusanli), which are known to increase energy and immunity. Next, place acupuncture needles into points LI-4 and PC-6 (Neiguan) to improve energy flow and alleviate tension. During the reflexology session, concentrate on points associated with the adrenal glands, spleen, and kidneys, since they are important for energy generation and stress management. This holistic therapy strategy may assist to relieve CFS symptoms by addressing the underlying imbalances.

Massage Therapy

Massage therapy is the technique of manipulating muscles and tissues to reduce tension and promote relaxation. It may be used with hand reflexology for a more complete and successful therapy. This combination treats both the muscular and reactive components of the body, improving overall health.

Combining Techniques:

Begin the session with a full-body massage to relax the client's muscles and get them ready for reflexology. This first massage relieves physical stress and improves circulation, making the body more amenable to reflexology therapy. Concentrate on regions that are very tight or painful, and use methods like kneading, stroking, and friction to relax the muscles and increase blood flow.

Hand and Arm Massage:

Use hand and arm massage methods to improve the reflexology session. Use wide, sweeping strokes on the arms to relax the muscles and enhance circulation. Pay specific attention to your forearms, which may get quite tense from repeated tasks like typing or physical labor. Massaging the hands and fingers may assist to relax the tiny muscles and joints, preparing them for more intense reflexology therapy.

Enhancing Reflexology Experience:

The combination of massage treatment with reflexology offers a comprehensive strategy that meets both musculoskeletal and reflexive demands. This massage relaxes the muscles and improves circulation, making them more susceptible to reflexology. Reflexology, in turn, helps to balance the body's systems and promotes general well-being, which enhances the advantages of massage.

Creating Synergistic Effects:

To have a synergistic impact, alternating massage and reflexology treatments during the session. For example, after massaging an individual's shoulders and arms, go to the hands and apply reflexology on the relevant reflex spots. This method helps to keep the person relaxed and improves the entire therapeutic experience.

Case Study for Carpal Tunnel Syndrome:

Using a case study of someone who has carpal tunnel syndrome (CTS). This ailment results from pressure on the median nerve in the wrist, which causes pain, numbness, and paralysis in the hand. A combination of massage treatment and reflexology may be very beneficial in relieving symptoms and encouraging healing.

Begin by massaging the forearms and hands with kneading and friction to relax the muscles and increase circulation. Pay specific attention to the wrists, utilizing moderate stretches and rotations to relieve tension and improve flexibility. During the reflexology session, concentrate on the reflex points for the wrist, forearm, and hand. This involves the base of the thumb and the middle of the palm, which may reduce pressure on the median nerve and facilitate recovery.

Massage and reflexology may be used alternately to treat both the muscle and neurological elements of CTS. The massage relaxes the muscles and relieves tension in the forearm and wrist, whilst reflexology activates the body's natural healing processes and restores equilibrium in the damaged regions. This comprehensive strategy may considerably improve symptoms and the client's overall quality of life.

Long-term Benefits:

Regular massage improves muscular flexibility, reduces chronic tension, and promotes general comfort. When paired with reflexology, it may boost the body's inherent capacity to heal and maintain equilibrium. Individuals who undergo frequent combination treatments may have increased circulation, lower stress levels, and general well-being and health.

Mindfulness & Meditation

Mindfulness and meditation activities may greatly improve the hand reflexology experience by encouraging mental and emotional equilibrium. These activities include concentrating the attention and being totally present in the moment, which may enhance the therapeutic benefits of reflexology.

Guided Meditation:

Start the reflexology treatment with a brief guided meditation to assist the client relax and become present. This may include coaching the person through deep breathing exercises and visualization strategies to relax the mind and body. A basic guided meditation can include imagining a quiet location, such as a beach or a forest, and urging the client to concentrate on their breath and bodily sensations.

Mindful breathing:

Encourage the person to concentrate on their breathing throughout the reflexology treatment. Deep, deliberate breathing may aid to increase relaxation and serenity. Instruct the client to take slow, deep breaths, inhaling deeply with the nose and holding for a time before releasing slowly through the mouth. This exercise may assist to relieve stress and provide a more peaceful experience.

Mindful Practices:

Mindfulness techniques may be included into reflexology sessions to boost their therapeutic effects. Encourage the client to exercise mindfulness by focusing on the sensations in their hands and body during the session. This might include observing the practitioner's hand pressure and motions, the warmth of the touch, and the spread of calm throughout the body. Focusing on the present moment allows the client to become more aware of their body and the healing process.

Combining With Reflexology:

Combining mindfulness and meditation with hand reflexology results in a comprehensive approach that addresses the physical, emotional, and mental components of wellness. Mindfulness activities assist to quiet the mind and increase the relaxation response, making reflexology more effective. Reflexology, in turn, may assist to balance the body's systems by providing a synergistic effect that amplifies the advantages of both techniques.

Case Study: Anxiety and Stress.

Examine a case study of a client with persistent anxiety and stress. This client might benefit greatly from the combination of mindfulness and meditation with hand reflexology. Begin the session with a guided meditation to assist the client relax and be present. Use visualization methods to take the client to a serene state, urging them to concentrate on their breath and bodily sensations.

Encourage the client to breathe mindfully and focus on the feelings in their hands and body throughout the reflexology treatment. Concentrate on reflex points related to the neurological system, such as brain and spinal cord reflex points in the fingers and thumb. This combination approach may assist to quiet the mind, decrease anxiety, and increase general relaxation.

Developing a Safe and Calm Environment:

The setting in which the reflexology session takes place is critical in maximizing the effects of mindfulness and meditation. Ensure that the therapy space is quiet, pleasant, and distraction-free. Soft lighting, quiet music, and a comfortable treatment table or chair may all contribute to a tranquil and pleasant setting. Encourage the client to withdraw from technological gadgets and concentrate only on the session.

Regular use of these approaches may help individuals develop better self-awareness, decrease stress, and enhance their overall mental and emotional health. Individuals may discover that they can better handle stress and anxiety over time, resulting in a higher quality of life.

Advanced Mindfulness Techniques:

More sophisticated approaches may be used in a reflexology session by those who have expertise with mindfulness and meditation. Body scanning techniques, in which the person deliberately concentrates on various regions of their body to relieve stress, are especially helpful. Guided imagery, in which the user imagines happy and healing pictures, may also improve the therapeutic benefits of reflexology. These advanced methods may assist enhance the relaxation response and increase feelings of well-being.

Finally, combining hand reflexology with other therapeutic methods including aromatherapy, acupressure, acupuncture, massage therapy, and mindfulness and meditation may dramatically improve treatment efficacy. Each modality has distinct advantages that, when combined with reflexology, provide a potent synergy that addresses the physical, emotional, and mental components of wellness.

Aromatherapy uses essential oils to improve the sensory experience and encourage relaxation. Acupressure and acupuncture use focused stimulation to regulate energy flow and facilitate healing. Massage treatment relaxes muscles and enhances circulation, making them more susceptible to reflexology. Mindfulness and meditation assist to quiet the mind and increase the relaxation response, making reflexology more effective.

By learning these complementing skills, you may provide a profoundly transforming reflexology experience that meets the requirements of the whole individual. Individuals who include these practices may see significant changes in their physical, emotional, and mental health, resulting in a better quality of life and a stronger feeling of balance and harmony.

Practitioners that take the effort to study and incorporate complementary therapies into their reflexology practice will be able to provide more effective and individualized treatments. The comprehensive approach will assist individuals by allowing them to relax deeper, relieve symptoms more effectively, and enhance their general well-being. This integrated approach to hand reflexology symbolizes the future of holistic health care, offering a complete and effective method for promoting healing and maintaining balance in the body, mind, and spirit.

CHAPTER 10.

SELF-CARE AND MAINTENANCE

Including self-care and maintenance techniques in your daily routine is critical for preserving the health and effectiveness of your hands. Hand reflexology may be an effective tool not just for others, but also for practitioners themselves. You may keep your hands in tip-top shape by practicing self-reflexology methods on a regular basis, following daily hand care suggestions, and conducting exercises to improve flexibility and strength.

Self-reflexology Techniques:

Self-reflexology enables you to receive the advantages of reflexology without the need for a practitioner. It's a handy approach to manage stress, alleviate pain, and live a better life. Start by locating a quiet, comfortable area where you can concentrate on your hands. Begin with deep breathing techniques to relax your mind and body. Inhale deeply through your nose, hold for a few seconds before gently exhaling through your mouth. This will help you relax and prepare for your reflexology treatment.

Begin your reflexology session with a gentle hand massage. Use a mild, soothing lotion or oil to make the motions smoother and more pleasant. Begin with wide, sweeping strokes over your palms, fingers, and wrists to relax the muscles and increase circulation. Pay extra attention to any tight or painful regions, kneading them gently with your thumb and fingers to relieve stress.

Next, concentrate on the reflex spots in your hands. Use your thumb to stroll down the diaphragm line, which is positioned just below the base of your fingers. Apply consistent pressure to this line as you go from one side of your palm to another. This method stimulates the reflex points and promotes general equilibrium. Move to the top portion of your hand and use both thumb and finger walking methods to activate response spots for your lungs and heart. To trigger reflex points in your stomach, liver, and pancreas, apply firm pressure to the center of your hand while walking with your thumb. These principles are critical to supporting gut health and metabolic function.

For the thumb, employ point pressing on the base to treat the neck reflex point, followed by the thumb walking down the length of the thumb to cover the head reflex points. Pay close attention to the pad of your thumb, which depicts the pituitary gland. This helps to relieve stress and tension in the head and neck regions.

Work on each finger by moving your finger from the base to the tip. The index finger represents the teeth and sinuses, the middle finger the brain, the ring finger the eyes and ears, and the little finger the shoulders and limbs. This complete stimulation aids in treating a variety of physiological processes.

Finally, travel to your wrist, which has reflex points for your lower back and intestines. To activate these points, use rotation and hooking methods while applying firm pressure to the wrist's inner and outer margins. This guarantees thorough covering and treats digestive and lower back issues.

Self-reflexology may help you manage stress, ease pain, and maintain good health. It's a simple yet powerful approach to include the advantages of reflexology into your everyday routine.

Daily Hand Care Tips:

Taking care of your hands on a regular basis is important, particularly for people who use them often in their work or personal lives. Here are some ways to maintain your hands healthy and functional:

1. Keep your hands moisturized by using a high-quality hand lotion or cream. Dry hands may crack and become uncomfortable, making reflexology and other duties difficult to do. Use lotion many times each day, particularly after washing your hands.

2. Protect your hands from the harsh environment. Wear gloves while cleaning, gardening, or doing any other activity that may expose your hands to chemicals, dirt, or severe temperatures. This prevents skin damage and protects the health of your hands.

3. Wash your hands with gentle soap and lukewarm water. Avoid using hot water and strong soaps, since they might deplete your skin's natural oils, causing dryness and irritation. Instead of rubbing, pat your hands dry with a soft cloth.

4. Keep your nails clipped and tidy. Smooth any rough edges using a nail file and don't bite or pick at your cuticles. Regular manicures may assist to maintain healthy nails and cuticles, lowering the chance of infection.

5. Include hand workouts in your everyday regimen to maintain strength and flexibility. Simple exercises, like creating a fist and then spreading your fingers wide, can help maintain your hands in excellent shape. Stretching your fingers, wrists and palms can also help avoid stiffness and increase range of motion.

6. Give your hands a regular massage to boost circulation and ease strain. Knead the palm, finger, and wrist muscles with your thumb and fingers. This may be done with or without lotion, and it is particularly helpful after a long day of using your hands.

7. Be aware of tasks that strain your hands and take frequent pauses to relax them. If you do repetitive chores, such as typing or using tools, be sure to take pauses and extend your hands to avoid strain and injury.

Exercises to Increase Hand Flexibility and Strength

Maintaining hand flexibility and strength is critical for successful reflexology practice and general hand health. Regular exercise may help avoid stiffness, increase dexterity, and strengthen your hands. Here are some activities to include into your routine:

Finger stretches: Extend your arm forward, palm facing up. Stretch the muscles in your forearm by gently pulling back on your fingers with your opposite hand. Hold this stretch for a few seconds, then move to the other hand. This exercise improves flexibility in your fingers and wrists.

Finger Lifts: Lay your hand flat on a table or another firm surface. Lift one finger at a time and hold it aloft for a few seconds before lowering it back down. Repeat this exercise with each finger, and then with the opposite hand. Finger lifts serve to develop the muscles in your fingertips while also improving coordination.

Fist Clenching: Make a fist with your hand and squeeze firmly for a few seconds. Then, open your hand and spread your fingers as much as possible. Repeat the exercise many times with each hand. Fist clenching and spreading assist to strengthen and stretch your hands and fingers.

Thumb Touches: Place the tip of your thumb against the tip of each finger, one at a time. This practice, known as "opposition," improves your thumb's dexterity and range of motion. Repeat the exercise many times with each hand.

Grip Strengthening: Use a stress ball or a tiny, soft ball to increase your grip strength. Squeeze the ball firmly, hold for a few seconds, and then release. Repeat the exercise many times with each hand. Grip-strengthening exercises are very effective in increasing total hand strength and endurance.

Wrist Rotations: Move your wrists in circular movements, starting clockwise and ending counterclockwise. This exercise promotes flexibility and mobility in your wrist joints, avoiding stiffness and improving range of motion.

Tendon Gliding: Place your hand flat on a table and raise each finger separately, keeping the others flat. This exercise increases the mobility and flexibility of the tendons in your hand. Repeat this exercise with each finger on both hands.

Adopting these self-care and maintenance routines into your daily routine can help keep your hands healthy, flexible, and strong. Regular self-reflexology sessions, regular hand care, and focused exercises can help you preserve your hands' functioning and well-being, enabling you to continue practicing reflexology and get the myriad advantages it provides. Whether you are a practitioner or just someone who loves the health of their hands, these activities are critical for long-term hand health.

CHAPTER 11

CASE STUDIES & TESTIMONIALS

Real-Life Case Studies

To properly comprehend the impact and efficiency of hand reflexology, it is necessary to review real-life case studies that show its therapeutic effects. These case studies give a thorough look at how hand reflexology can be used to treat a variety of health concerns and the outcomes that can be obtained.

Case Study 1: Relieving Chronic Headaches

Jane, a 35-year-old lady, has been experiencing terrible headaches for more than a decade. Despite attempting a variety of treatments, including pharmaceutical and other therapies, she received no cure. After seeing a reflexologist, she decided to try hand reflexology. The practitioner began by completing a lengthy procedure on Jane's hands, concentrating on reflex spots related to the head and neck. Over many weeks, Jane observed a dramatic decrease in the frequent and severe headaches. By stimulating certain reflex areas on her hands, the practitioner was able to relieve the tension and stress that were causing her headaches. Jane's story demonstrates the potential of hand reflexology to decrease chronic pain issues.

Case Study 2: Managing Stress and Anxiety.

Mark, a 45-year-old businessman, felt a lot of stress and worry because of his demanding job. He battled with sleeplessness and had difficulty relaxing. Mark sought a comprehensive approach to stress management and resorted to hand reflexology. The practitioner concentrated on reflex points connected to the adrenal glands, heart and solar plexus, which are known to affect stress and anxiety. After many sessions, Mark reported feeling more calm and capable of managing his stress. He also observed better sleep quality. This instance highlights how hand reflexology may help manage stress and anxiety while also increasing general well-being.

Case Study 3: Promoting Digestive Health

Sarah, a 50-year-old lady, suffers from persistent digestive problems like bloating, constipation, and gas. Traditional therapies offered little help, so she decided to try hand reflexology. The reflexologist focused on reflex spots on Sarah's hands that corresponded to her stomach, intestines, and liver. Sarah's gut health improved significantly throughout many sessions. Her bloating went down, her bowel motions became more regular, and she felt more comfortable overall. This instance demonstrates how hand reflexology may improve digestive health by activating reflex sites associated with the digestive organs.

Success Stories for Practitioners and Clients

Success stories from both practitioners and customers demonstrate the transformational potential of hand reflexology. These testimonials give useful information about the various applications and advantages of this holistic therapy.

The Practitioner's Perspective

Ann, a seasoned reflexologist, has seen many success stories in her profession. One of her most notable cases was with a lady who had significant arthritis in her hands. Mary had discomfort and stiffness, which limited her ability to complete everyday duties. Ann, tailored a hand reflexology program for Mary's requirements, concentrating on reflex spots associated with the joints and immune system. Mary gradually felt less discomfort and had more movement in her hands. Ann's ability to tailor the reflexology routine to her client's health and demands demonstrates the adaptability and efficacy of hand reflexology in addressing chronic diseases.

The Client's Perspective

John, a 60-year-old retired teacher, discusses his experience with hand reflexology. He had been suffering from chronic weariness and poor energy levels for some years. After learning about reflexology from a friend, John decided to try it. To increase his energy levels, the practitioner concentrated on reflex points associated with the adrenal glands, thyroid, and solar plexus. John noted a progressive rise in his energy and stamina after several sessions. He felt more balanced and refreshed. John's experience demonstrates how hand reflexology may assist in boosting energy and improving quality of life.

Common Challenges and Ways to Overcome Them

While hand reflexology can provide several advantages, practitioners, and consumers may face certain problems. Understanding these problems and how to overcome them is critical for achieving good results.

Initial Discomfort:

Some persons may feel discomfort during their first few reflexology treatments, particularly if they have sensitive or stiff reflex sites. To address this, practitioners should begin with light pressure and gradually raise the intensity as the client grows used to the therapy. Effective communication between the practitioner and the client is critical for ensuring comfort and addressing any problems quickly.

Consistency and Commitment:

Significant benefits with hand reflexology generally need constant and frequent sessions. Some customers may struggle to keep a consistent program owing to time restrictions or a lack of rapid results. Educating clients on the long-term advantages of frequent reflexology sessions might help them commit. Offering flexible scheduling choices and follow-up reminders can also help customers stay on track with their treatments.

Managing Expectations:

Clients may have different expectations for the results of hand reflexology. treatment is critical for practitioners to convey accurate information about what reflexology may do and how long treatment may take to produce benefits. Setting specific goals and clarifying the holistic nature of reflexology can assist to moderate expectations and build a productive therapeutic relationship.

Addressing Specific Health Conditions:

While hand reflexology can benefit a variety of health disorders, it may not be a one-stop treatment for all problems. Integrating reflexology with other therapeutic modalities and conventional therapies can boost its efficacy. Practitioners should be familiar with various health issues and know when to send patients to other healthcare providers for complete care.

Practice Self-Care:

As a hand reflexology practitioner, you may experience physical strain or burnout as a result of their regular practice. To address this, you can practice self-care by adding hand and wrist exercises, keeping proper ergonomics and taking frequent breaks. Using tools and assistance can also help lessen physical strain and ensure long-term success in their profession.

Examining real-life case studies, sharing success stories and addressing frequent difficulties lead to a thorough grasp of hand reflexology's effect and potential. These findings show the adaptability of hand reflexology in treating a variety of health issues, boosting general well-being and improving quality of life. By learning from these experiences, both practitioners and clients can optimize the advantages of hand reflexology while overcoming any hurdles that may arise. Mastery in hand reflexology necessitates not just technical abilities but also empathy, communication and a complete approach to healthiness. Practitioners can also provide transformational and therapeutic experiences to their clients via devotion and constant study, making hand reflexology an important component of complete health care.

CHAPTER 12

HOW TO BECOME A PROFESSIONAL REFLEXOLOGIST

Training And Certification Requirements

Beginning the road to becoming a professional reflexologist requires a dedication to learning, skill development, and professional certification. The first step is to receive extensive instruction from a reputable school. Reflexology programs are offered by a variety of institutions and training institutes across the world, and they address both theoretical knowledge and practical skills. These programs often include substantial hands-on practice, an in-depth study of human anatomy and physiology, as well as the history and concepts of reflexology.

Choosing the appropriate training program is essential. Look for approved schools that adhere to the criteria established by professional reflexology groups. Accreditation assures that the training is of high quality and recognized by the industry. Courses should provide a balanced curriculum that includes both classroom and supervised practical activities. Instructors should be seasoned practitioners who can offer helpful advice and mentoring.

After completing the training program, the next step is to gain certification. Certification criteria vary by nation and area but they often include passing a written test and proving practical ability. In the United States, for example, the American Reflexology Certification Board (ARCB) administers a national certification test. This accreditation is highly recognized and can help you establish credibility as a practitioner. Other nations have their certification bodies, such as the Association of Reflexologists (AoR) in the United Kingdom and the Reflexology Association of Canada (RAC).

Continuing education is a vital part of professional growth. Reflexology is a dynamic subject that is always expanding via study and techniques. Staying up to speed on the newest advances through workshops, seminars and advanced courses can not only improve your abilities but also keep you competitive in the industry.

Building Your Practice:

Once qualified, establishing a successful reflexology practice necessitates strategic preparation and a dedication to quality. Begin by developing a business strategy including your objectives, target market, services provided, price and marketing tactics. This plan will serve as a road map for your practice, allowing you to keep focused on your goals.

Finding the appropriate place is another crucial factor. Whether you operate from a home office, a wellness center or a specialized clinic, make sure the setting is calm, pleasant and relaxing. The area should be outfitted with the required equipment and resources, such as a comfortable chair or table, reflexology charts and hygiene items.

Networking is also a crucial part of growing your practice. Join professional organizations like the International Institute of Reflexology (IIR) and the Reflexology Association of America. These organizations provide invaluable information, networking opportunities and reputation. Attend industry conferences and workshops to meet other professionals, share ideas and learn about the newest trends and techniques.

Providing excellent customer service is important for keeping customers and earning recommendations. Make sure every client feels satisfied and cared for from the time they come in touch with you. Listen to their needs, offer individualized therapies and follow up to monitor their progress. Building great relationships with your clients will result in recurring business and favourable word-of-mouth recommendations.

Ethical Concerns and Professionalism

As a reflexologist, keeping high ethical standards and professionalism is essential. Adhere to an ethical code that puts your clients' well-being and dignity first. Confidentiality is critical; always safeguard your clients' personal and medical information.

Informed consent is another key component of ethical behaviour. Before beginning therapy, clearly explain the reflexology process to your customers, including the advantages and any potential concerns. Ensure that they comprehend and accept the treatment plan.

Boundaries must be followed at all times. Maintain a professional manner and avoid any actions that may be construed as unprofessional. This involves physical limits, such as touching only pertinent regions during therapy, as well as emotional boundaries, such as refraining from pushing personal views or attitudes on clients.

Professionalism also includes your appearance and demeanour. Dress correctly, practice decent personal cleanliness and foster a pleasant and professional atmosphere. Punctuality is also vital; honour your clients' time by beginning and concluding meetings on time.

Continuous self-assessment and development are required to retain professionalism. Regularly solicit input from clients and coworkers to find areas for improvement. Engage in reflective practice to identify your strengths and places for improvement.

Marketing and Growing Your Customer Base

Effective marketing is critical for acquiring and maintaining customers. Begin by building a professional website that showcases your skills, qualifications and contact information. Include customer testimonials and case studies to increase credibility and demonstrate the advantages of reflexology.

Use social media tools to reach a larger audience. Share educational reflexology content, such as articles, videos and customer success stories. Engage your audience by replying to comments and inquiries, and utilize targeted advertising to reach out to local clients.

Networking with other healthcare professionals might also help you build a customer base. Develop relationships with chiropractors, massage therapists, acupuncturists and other complementary health professionals. These specialists can suggest clients to you and vice versa, resulting in a mutually beneficial network.

Offering workshops and seminars is another great strategy to promote your practice. Educate the community on the benefits of reflexology by conducting free or low-cost workshops. This not only exhibits your knowledge but also allows potential clients to try out your services firsthand.

Special promos and bundles can entice new customers and increase repeated purchases. Provide discounts to first-time clients, referral bonuses or bundle packages for several sessions. These incentives might help you establish a loyal clientele and produce consistent revenue.

In conclusion, being a professional reflexologist entails extensive training, certification and ongoing professional growth. Building a successful practice involves strategic planning, networking and outstanding customer service. Adhering to ethical norms and being professional are critical for establishing trust and confidence. Effective marketing and community participation will help you expand your clientele and build a flourishing practice. By committing to quality in all aspects of your work, you will succeed as a professional reflexologist and make a significant impact on your client's health status.